Affirmations for Black Men
Overcome Self-Sabotage, Boost Your Self-Esteem,
Confidence, and
Attract Success by Reprogramming Your Mind with
Positive Affirmations

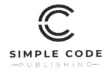

SIMPLE CODE
—PUBLISHING—

Printed or published to the highest ethical standard

Affirmations for Black Men

By Nathen Hughes

United States
2022

CONTENTS

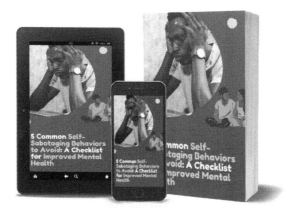

A FREE GIFT TO OUR READERS

5 Common Self-Sabotaging Behaviors to Avoid
downloadable guideline.

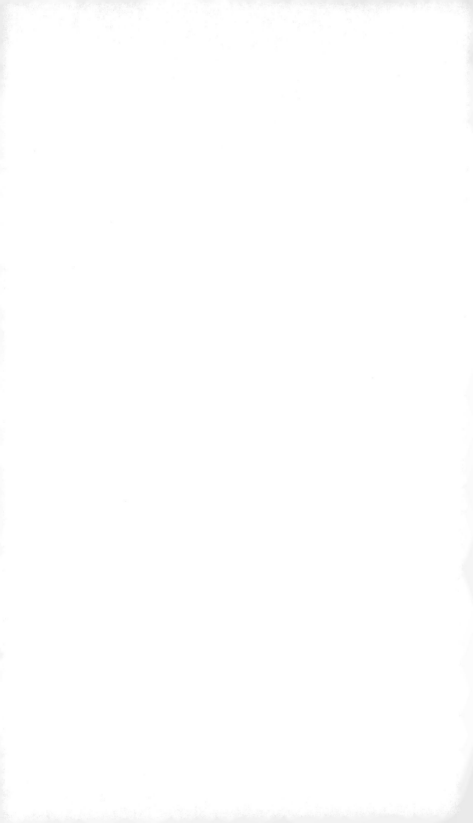

INTRODUCTION: WHAT DOES IT MEAN TO BE A BLACK MAN TODAY?

The meaning of masculinity in the United States and how it is evolving has been a topic of discussion. Additionally, for some black males, the answer has little to do with gender and everything to do with race. How do you define being a black man? Luckily for our listeners we have interviewed a hand full of black men in the major cities, these are there responses.

"We have a lot of brains. Now that we've finished school, we're well-informed. We are optimistic, you know. Aspirations exist within us. As a team, we are working toward something. All of us value family time."

"It's hard to get hired, hard to find a place to live, hard to make ends meet in such a racist country."

"Today's racism is extremely complex. It's all very subtle, but they definitely make it clear that you're black. Oh, you have rasta dreads; you have this; you have that; therefore, you are this. Then, when I open my mouth, people are stunned. You use a unique language. I refuse to take any of that on myself. The burden of responsibility for that lies with that individual."

"When I left home to join the military, I finally felt like a man. When I had to stand up for my rights as a black man when applying for a job, I knew I was a black man. Obviously, I'm mentally capable. And I do possess a soul."

"Personally, I've experienced racial profiling in Brooklyn. I was on my way to the corner store to pick up an Arizona iced tea when I was stopped by five white police officers."

"I am 138 pounds and 5 feet, 8 inches tall. The officers then placed me in handcuffs and led me downstairs to the station. For what reason, I inquired. They never gave me a reason. My faith was dashed when I realized that we couldn't rely on the people who are supposed to be guarding us. On the other hand, they are responsible for our deaths."

"Imagine yourself in my position for a moment. Envision yourself on a walk down the street when someone crosses the street to avoid you because you are a black man. Picture this: you're walking down the street, when a police officer pulls you over and frisks you because you're black or because of what you're wearing. Put yourself in his shoes if he were your son. Consider that person your cousin, your brother, or your nephew. Try to picture that and then, you know, try to make sense of what we're going through, because it's tough. The going is rough."

"And as a black man, I'm trying to follow my own advice: don't give up the fight. Don't give up, no matter how tempting it is to do so. Just wait until tomorrow, because it's going to be another day."

"To me, being a black man means that I am respected and feared everywhere I go. That's fit for a king. In the end, I will reign supreme."

As you can see, it's tough being a black man, this is why we need affirmations to reprogram our minds counter against all odds.

When it comes to transitioning from one day to the next, affirmations are crucial. Affirmations serve as a constant reminder to keep going, even on the bad days. More importantly, they serve as a constant reminder that you are worthy of good things in life despite your shortcomings.

Do you want to change your way of thinking and make progress? If so, I hope these affirmations below will be of some use to you.

You can read one every day, or you can read them all at once. It's only through repeated exposure that you'll come to accept them as true, so let's get started!

Three Easy Ways to Incorporate Affirmations Into Your Daily Routine
1. Inhale deeply.
2. Affirm your positive affirmation aloud.
    While you are saying the affirmation, also:
    See yourself as you would like to be, complete with the qualities you seek (perhaps more self-assurance). your focus on what you know you can do well). Try shutting your eyes if that helps.

Express your desired emotions by repeating your affirmation, SPEAK AS IF YOU BELIEVE THAT AFFIRMATIVELY

3. Now is the time to reflect on how wonderful you currently feel.
Finally, that's all there is to it!

Affirmations of positivity are easy to use.

Don't forget the two crucial elements, though, that make them so powerful:

a) Feel the good vibes in your body by affirming them
b) Repetition is key.

AFFIRMATIONS

1. I know I can make it through today; in the end, it's how I approach challenges that will determine how much stress I end up under.

2. The macho role doesn't require constant performance on my part. Being a sensitive man has helped me avoid hurting anyone's feelings by alerting me to the times when I've been too harsh.

3. I've learned that development is a continuous process because I am a work in progress. There is always room for improvement. There's always room for improvement in my performance. You can always count on me for assistance.

4. The trivial actions of others need not have the consequential effect they sometimes do on my life.

5. Both today and tomorrow are days on which I need not be flawless. After all, there is no such thing as a perfect human being, not at work, in the gym, or anywhere else.

6. During my workout today, I plan to challenge myself a little bit more than usual. I plan to work out until I know I've given it my all.

7. No matter what difficulties today may bring, I will face them head-on like the man I am and do everything in my power to find the most effective ways to overcome them.

8. It is important that I exist. To me, my beliefs are critical. My opinion counts.

9. And I certainly am not wasting my time. It doesn't matter what you need, I'm here for you. I have no interest in leaving this world before I have lived to the fullest.

10. The decisions I make have far-reaching consequences, but I'm confident I'm making the best ones.

11. A former me enjoyed making a good impression on others. At this point in my life, I enjoy proving my worth to myself, and I take great pride in the man I've become so far.

12. I am not bolstered by compliments. Competence is what gives me faith in myself.

13. Only by altering my own perspective can I bring about a revolution in society.

14. To me, my wife is nothing less than a queen. My little boys and girls are the princes and princesses of my heart. I must remember that in their eyes I am a king and act accordingly.

15. Nothing is worse than someone who is a doormat. I have no problem assisting others, but I won't put up with being pushed around.

16. I have discovered the meaning of respect by showing it to myself even when others do not.

17. I can try to fill my head with ideas of where to go, but I'll never find my true north or my life's purpose unless I first look within.

18. When I'm sick, my health is the most important thing to me. How healthy I am is entirely under my control, as my body is mine.

19. I don't care what other people think of me because I know that my life is progressing in the right direction for me.

20. As I progress in my career, I hope to improve my current performance.

21. Supercharging Your Life With Positive Affirmations for Men I am doing well in my career and will continue to learn how to do even better. | daily affirmations | affirmations to improve mental health | affirmations for men in pdf format

22. Some people pick up on my affable vibe and it motivates them to see the value in staying optimistic.

23. It's only fair that life treats me well. Mistakes are just that, and I've grown as a result of my own.

24. I can show joy when I am happy, sadness when I am sad, gratitude when I am thankful, and humor when I am humorous.

25. When I talk about my ideas with other people, we can make a difference.

26. My life seems to draw me toward accomplishment, and I've found that there are countless paths to financial success.

27. Even if you and I have different standards for what constitutes success, we are both successful in our own ways.

28. When I use my special skills to help others, the world will be a better place.

29. Because I am deserving of joy, I am surrounded by joy, laughter, peace, and abundance.

30. Recognizing my own shortcomings and admitting my ignorance are essential components of growing as a person.

31. I do not just exist without purpose in this world. The world is a better place because of me, and I know that.

32. To what extent I am accountable to others is a decision that must be made by me, and I have come to the realization that I am accountable to no one but myself.

33. Whether I zoom out to see the big picture or in on the finer details, I always see how vital I am.

34. Supercharging Your Life with Positive Affirmations for Men I am valuable whether I consider the big picture or the details only. #men #positiveaffirmations #dailyaffirmations | affirmations for husbands | affirmations for men | affirmations for black men

35. When I am confronted with ambiguity, I know that it exists for a purpose.

36. In today's world, I will not be a failure.

37. The keys to my success, or failure, lie in my own hands.

38. I have the fortitude and skill to overcome any obstacle I face.

39. I'm living my life with a sense of purpose, and it's filled me with enthusiasm, vitality, and satisfaction. It is with this goal in mind that I have taken up the challenge of life.

40. Insofar as I take care of myself and listen to my inner voice, I won't need any other guidance.

41. I have confidence in my looks and can bring myself to smile every day. I can enhance my physical appearance by depending on my own resources, working hard, and making consistent efforts.

42. In my experience, the connections I've made have been both positive and productive. When I'm around my friends and coworkers, I feel supported and encouraged. I can validate who I am apart from the approval of naysayers.

43. I am comfortable striking up conversations with strangers and have the confidence to do so. The more people I meet, the more I feel like I have something to offer to the world.

44. I can look back with satisfaction on my accomplishments and confidently outline the next steps I took to get where I am today. I know this next step will be difficult, but my confidence in myself will see me through.

45. I am confident in my abilities and derive pleasure from surprising people.

46. I can teach myself anything if I put in the effort. When I give myself enough time, I can learn as much as I need to about a problem before attempting to solve it.

47. Having confidence in myself does not rely solely on the opinions of others.

48. Affirmations for men: I do not need the approval of others to feel good about myself. Affirmations for a man's health | positive words to live by | words to encourage a man's spirit

49. There is a process involved in gaining wisdom from past errors, and I recognize that. I have made some errors in judgment and am working to correct them.

50. I can overcome any obstacle because I am strong and courageous. I anticipate doing so daily, in fact.

51. The things I'm afraid of are nothing I can't handle. I used to do that.

52. Today is the day I make it. But if I don't succeed, I'll figure out what I did right in spite of my setbacks.

53. When I'm by myself, I can think quickly on my feet and come up with solutions without giving up any of who I am.

54. As a person, success is ingrained in me. I want to get a lot more done. The combination of ambition and self-control will ensure that I am never without the motivation to push myself further.

55. There has been too much progress for me to give up on my goals now. I have a clear plan for where to go and how to get there, as well as next steps for when I reach my objectives.

56. I thrive on taking on difficult tasks at which I know I will inevitably struggle. By challenging myself and exposing my weak spots, I am able to make progress toward my goals.

57. To a greater extent than my failures, I focus on my achievements. The truth is, though, that it is precisely my setbacks that have given me the strength to succeed.

58. In order to protect the people I care about, I possess tremendous bravery and will go to any lengths necessary.

59. When things get tough, I become even more focused on reaching my goals. I believe the more I share my experience, the more people will take something away from it.

60. I intend to keep striving to be the most capable man I can be by accepting accountability and placing value on the things that really matter. Instead of self-destructing for fun, I'd rather keep up with my commitments.

61. There are times when I am content with accepting second best because I know I am giving it my all and achieving the best results I can.

62. Affirmations for men: I know I am doing the best I can, so it's okay if I have to settle for less sometimes. Affirmations for the Day | Affirmations for Black Men | Affirmations for Alpha Males

63. 59.. When I make time for the things that I enjoy, I feel most like myself. I find more satisfaction in my life when my pursuits and passions allow me to make a global difference.

64. When a problem arises, I am prepared to handle it. In other words, I don't need to have it drilled into my head.

65. Those I care about have a high regard for me. As long as I maintain my integrity, I will continue to be accorded the respect for which I have become known.

66. I like to think and talk in a positive manner. Although I am far from perfect, I have learned that optimism, hope, and faith are the fuel that keep me going.

67. I'm able to poke fun at my own foibles and do so with relish. My personality is straightforward, and there are obvious benefits to spending time with me.

68. So long as I do what I need to, I'll be in a good place to flourish.

69. For many reasons, I adore myself. I am actively working to improve the aspects of myself that I do not currently appreciate.

70. For the most part, I have been successful.

71. Having said that, I am confident.

72. When I speak, people listen.
73. I am mighty.
74. It seems like every day I make some sort of improvement.
75. The resources I require are already within me.
76. When I first open my eyes in the morning, I feel inspired.

77. To put it simply, I am a tornado that can't be stopped.
78. My very existence serves as a demonstration of the power of inspiration.
79. This is a time of great prosperity for me.
80. The people I interact with are being uplifted and encouraged by me.
81. Through my work, I am able to encourage others.
82. I am not going to give in to the negative emotions or thoughts that have been trying to control my mind.
83. What a fantastic day it is today.
84. At the same time that I am turning up the positive in my life, I am turning down the negative.
85. My mind is laser-focused.
86. My problems don't drive me; my aspirations do.
87. I appreciate everything that God has provided for me.
88. I'm able to take care of myself and don't need anyone else.
89. What I am depends entirely on my own desires.
90. What motivates me is not my past, but rather my potential in the future.
91. The challenges I face push me to improve and broaden my horizons.
92. A lot of work will get done today.
93. Intelligent and determined best describe me.
94. Every day, my sense of gratitude grows.
95. The passing days have allowed me to gradually recover my health.
96. I am getting closer and closer to my objectives with each passing day.

97. Weird things are happening to me and around me right now, and it's all because of the power of my thoughts and words.
98. I am continually developing into a more admirable person.
99. I'm releasing all of the negative self-doubt and fear that's been holding me back.
100. By embracing my uniqueness, I am able to cultivate inner calm, strength, and self-assurance.
101. To set myself free, I must first forgive myself. In return for your forgiveness, please forgive me.
102. Day by day, I feel better and stronger.
103. In the past, I have overcome adversity and emerged from it better and stronger for it. And yet, I know that I can get through this.
104. Not a single day of my life goes to waste. I make the most of every moment of today, tomorrow, and every day of my life.
105. Keep in mind the tremendous strength I have within me to accomplish anything.
106. If someone or something isn't good for me, I don't give them the chance to inject harmful ideas and thoughts into my head; instead, I cut ties and move on.
107. I have a place here, and I am valued by those who know me.
108. Even though I have a dreadful history, I am a stunning woman now.
109. Mistakes I've made are not who I am.
110. My inner glow warms the hearts of those around me.

111.   I try not to judge myself against others. My only standard of comparison is yesterday's self. I consider myself successful if the person I am today is even a little bit better than the person I was yesterday.

112.   To myself: You will be so proud of me.

113.   I complete the tasks at hand and let the rest go.

114.   When I eat, it's like a meal for my soul. In order to strengthen my body, I exercise regularly. I force myself to concentrate. Okay, now is my turn.

115.   There is a purpose to my existence. The work that I do matters. My deeds have depth and can motivate others.

116.   I've done all I could with the resources I had today. And I am grateful for that opportunity.

117.   Just one upbeat thought first thing in the morning can set the tone for the entire day. So, I'm starting my day off right by thinking a positive, motivating thought that will echo success throughout the rest of my day.

118.   I make plans and pursue them with every ounce of grit I possess. The places I go when I do this are only limited by my own abilities and skills.

119.   Today, I make the conscious decision to feel joy.

120.   I don't need to lower my standards or change who I am to please or appease anyone who is not willing to accept me for what I am.

121.   Nothing about me, including the color of my skin, can determine whether or not I have a place in this world.

122.   accept being able to ignore my presence or mute my voice because of the color of my skin.

123.   If there is anyone in my life who attempts to upset or negatively impact me, I will remove them from my orbit and replace them with upbeat, supportive people.

124.   disturb me, I will kindly exclude them from my immediate vicinity so that I can return my attention to the

125.   spirit beings with whom I have a deep emotional bond.

126.   I'm allowed to feel human, and crying is one of those things.

127.   and to grieve, to feel disappointment, to feel shame, to make mistakes, to fail, to laugh, and to cry.

128.   sing my praises, and I'll finally be able to fully embrace my humanity and bask in all its splendor.

129.   As a dwelling place for God, my physical form is nothing short of a work of art.

130.   I am a product of the skill of his hands.

131. The sun's rays have touched my skin, and I feel slightly warmer as a result.

132. In a sky full of stars, I stand out as Polaris; my presence will be honored; I am revered.

133. Rather than being another discarded black body, you should refuse to be one.

134. I will give myself permission to change and grow; I will have faith in my method and give myself credit for my achievements.

135. I am trying, and I will accept that as sufficient.

136. Even though I am not perfect, I am aware of my many redeeming features.

137. Excellence in both aesthetics and learning. Never again will I allow my doubts to overshadow my value.

138. Because I am respectful, kind, and loving toward others, and because I have a strong sense of integrity, I deserve respect.

139. I'm going to make it anyway.

140. I will not give in to my foes; rather, I will remain true to my principles and refuse to compromise.

141. This self-love I cultivate will be the source of peace in my life.

142. For as long as I live, I intend to take the measures necessary to ensure that I have the best possible chance of living a happy, successful, and fulfilled life.

143. No matter what comes my way, I will not be uprooted from the solid foundation of selfless love.

144. I will never doubt my abilities or diminish my expectations of myself.

145. I accept and appreciate myself just the way I am.

146. When it comes to my own judgment, I have complete faith in myself.

147. With each stride I take, I become more powerful.

148. Whatever I put my mind to, I will accomplish.

149. That I am powerful and capable.

150. No challenge is too great for me to overcome.

151. I take deep breaths of assurance and release my worries.

152. The emotion of fear is fleeting. I am able to take action despite anxiety.

153. By letting go of my doubt, I make way for success.

154. I'm not shy about talking to new people; in fact, I thrive on it.

155. When it comes to my own worth and beauty, I am completely satisfied.

156.   It's important to me to focus on the here and now, but I also have faith in the future.
157.   An air of self-assurance permeates everything I do.
158.   I like to think of myself as an outgoing and confident person.

159.   My independence, originality, and tenacity serve me well in any endeavor.
160.   I have a lot of vitality and excitement. I've always been a confident person.
161.   Everything that happens to me is for the best, and I only attract positive and happy experiences.
162.   I enjoy figuring out complicated issues and helping others do the same.
163.   By putting my mind to it, I always come up with the best
164.   solution.
165.   I am very adaptable, and I enjoy being thrust into unfamiliar situations.
166.   I thrive when tested. Because of them, I am able to shine brighter than I ever have before.
167.   Everything is within my reach.
168.   In order to succeed today, I am prepared to fail.
169.   I'm very pleased with my effort to even try this.
170.   I have taken good care of myself and can confidently say that I am healthy and well-groomed.

171. My health on the outside is paralleled by my internal peace.

172. I function best when I am assured of my own abilities. There is no such thing as an impossible task, and life is

173. great.

174. There is no bad in anyone else's eyes in mine.

175. Positive people are drawn to me.

176. I am confident and brave in the face of adversity.

177. When I need to find a solutions to these types of problems.

178. There are no conditions attached to my self-love and acceptance.

179. The world owes me a favor because I am a worthy human being.

180. In general, I like and approve of myself very highly.

181. Respect and adoration are returned to me in equal measure.

182. People really care about me and respect me.

183. Thanks to my lofty sense of self-worth, I am able to respect others and to be respected in return.

184. My goals are achievable because I am strong enough to achieve them.

185. It's up to me to decide what to do.

186. You should hold me in high regard because I am a one-of-a-kind, very special human being.

187. Everyday, I grow more and more fond of who I am as a person.

188. As a result of my healthy sense of self-worth, I am able to take compliments in stride.

189. When I accept people for who they are, they do the same for me.

190. What other people think is irrelevant. The only thing that matters is my response and my opinion.

191. When I give and receive love and acceptance, the world rewards me.

192. In order to fully enjoy the present, I have made the decision to let go of the past. As a result, I

193. get to take advantage of life to the fullest.

194. I value myself highly, so I feel good about myself.

195. That's right, I came out on top.

196. That which is good in the world is mine due.

197. There is no longer any requirement for your pain and anguish.

198. I let go of the need to prove myself to anyone because I am already complete and that's perfect for me!

199. I always try to find a workable answer.

200. There is always a way to deal with whatever issue arises.

201. I am never completely alone. Everything in the cosmos is on my side and rooting for me.

202. Thoughts of love, health, positivity, and success fill my head with ideas, which I then translate into actual events.

203. I am Incredibly blessed, my thoughts are filled with thanksgiving.

204. The choice to be self-assured is mine today and every day.

205. I radiate confidence, certainty and optimism

206. When presented with a chance, I don't hesitate to boldly push it open and take advantage of it.

207. Every aspect of my life is planned out by me.

208. I can make my dreams a reality.

209. Imagination is all I need to achieve anything.

210. I speak up for my convictions.

211. I take bold, sure steps.

212. I have faith in myself.

213. I like to think outside the norm and have an imaginative mind.

214. My thoughts and plans always end up well for me.

215. In the morning, I get up and do something that matters.

216. Every day, my company expands.

217. This thing I'm making is bigger than me.

218. Currently, I am living out my life's mission.

219. Forgive me, I utterly fail

220. No longer do I have to let my past define me; I get to make my own future from here on out.

221. I release my anger and hatred toward those who have wronged me.
222. Those who have wronged me in the past are forgiven, and I am at peace with myself again.
223. With all three, my life is abundant.
224. Each new door I walk through is replete with possibilities and benefits.
225. It seems that the more I give to others, the more they give back to me.
226. Current activities help me achieve my ultimate goals.
227. Anytime I want, I can instantly alter the way I'm thinking.
228. What I do with my life is entirely up to me.
229. It is within my control to make positive changes.
230. Having fun and enjoying life is something I allow myself to do.
231. Because of me, the world is better.
232. There is nothing that has happened or will happen that has upset me.
233. This is only the start of my life.
234. I'm making a conscious decision today to replace my negative routines with more constructive ones.
235. I'm so thankful that I was able to kick my vices.
236. I have finally broken my addictions.
237. I only engage in good routines.
238.
239. I am grateful for the opportunity to see another day.

240.   I have a colorful and lovely view of the world.

241.   Whatever good happens to me today is entirely deserved.

242.   There are many doors of possibility opening for me today, and I am ready to welcome them in.

243.   I make an effort to show my close friends how much they mean to me.

244.   The good things that happen to me are a direct result of the good vibes I put out into the world.

245.   I'm just chilling out and seeing where life takes me.

246.   Yes, I will choose joy today and every day.

247.   People enjoy being around me because I am lively and upbeat.

248.   The joy and love in my life are endless.

249.   Nothing ever stands in the way of my joy.

250.   Sustaining my mind with positive ideas is how I keep it going.

251.   Good nutrition is how I keep myself going.

252.   I fuel myself with nutritious foods.

253.   Exercising keeps my head and body fueled.

254.   In every way, my body is getting healthier by the day.

255.   I feel healthier and more energized by the day.

256.   I am a leader in every sense of the word.

257.   An Inspiring Leader Is Me

258.   Other people look up to me as a model

259.   I motivate people to become their best selves.

260. As a leader, I always try to set a good example.
261. I have the ability to convey my ideas clearly and concisely.
262. For as much as I love the world, it loves me right back.
263. I make the decision to share with others today and every day.
264. I make the decision to improve the world today, and every day.
265. I see love everywhere I turn.
266. My ideal companion is actively looking for me.
267. Sincerely, unconditionally, I love my partner.
268. I feel blessed to have found someone with whom to share this wonderful life.
269. As a result, my immediate circle is always full of cheery, supportive souls.
270. This is the day I might finally meet the one.
271. Ready for love: I am
272. Over time, my feelings for myself have only grown.
273. Both my family and my friends are incredible blessings in my life.
274. It never seems to be a problem for me to find adequate funds.
275. Money comes to me like a glistening river of gold.
276. Seeing my savings expand is a joy.
277. Many of my thoughts revolve around how to make a profit.
278. My salary keeps going up and up.

279. The amount of money I give away is always multiplied back to me.
280. Currently, I am laying claim to my portion.
281. I am blessed with a steady stream of income.
282. I have earned a comfortable lifestyle
283. I thrive on being pushed to my limits because it forces me to develop.
284. Every event in my life has taught me something and provided me with a chance to grow.
285.
286. Each day, my outlook becomes more positive and healthy.
287. My timing is impeccable, and I never miss a crucial opportunity.
288. I am equipped to handle this difficulty.
289. As a result of overcoming obstacles, I have grown as a person.
290. Every experience has helped me develop and expand.
291. The current events are working out for my highest good.
292. I've made a conscious effort to replace my bad routines with more productive ones.
293. Every day, I am able to accomplish more.
294. I am extremely self-disciplined, and that is why I will ultimately be successful.
295. Because I am willing to put in more effort than anyone else, I always come out on top.
296. I refuse to give up until it's my last breath.
297. I make efficient use of my time because I know how precious it is.

298. The work that I do is always disciplined and fruitful on my part.

299. I consider myself to be the most attractive person in my social circle.

300. In short, I'm a good person who wants to show the world how good my heart is.

301. I am currently in a position of complete autonomy in which to make a choice about my next course of action.

302. I was sent here as a present to the world.

303. I am special and have a lot to give to the world.

304. I am the epitome of sexiness.

305. I can decide whether to accept or reject an offer.

306. Daily, I make a conscious decision to focus on what really matters to me.

307. My decision to succeed today, and every day, is a conscious one.

308. I am not driven by desperation, but rather by inspiration when making decisions.

309. Good fortune and achievement seem to be drawn to me.

310. I've grown both physically and mentally since yesterday.

311. That's right, I'm a genius and I use my knowledge in my daily life.

312. Success-minded, like-minded people are drawn to me like a magnet.

313. I'm increasing in success every day, in every way.

314. Because of how I was raised, I always expect to be happy and successful.
315. A model of success and achievement, I am.
316. In every endeavor, I give my all and achieve the highest standards.
317. Possibilities and rewards abound in my exciting and thrilling life.
318. I will not stray from my path
319. Issues? I've got answers.
320. I am getting closer to my objectives every day, and especially today.
321. I have identified my higher purpose and am working toward it.
322. I have a job that matters and makes a difference in the world.
323. I'm willing to try new things.
324. I am the definition of success
325. I have earned my success.
326. Just being myself is the best option available.
327. That suffices for me.
328. Daily, I make more progress toward my goal.
329. My character is unparalleled.
330. Each of my issues can be fixed.
331. I am a leader now.
332. For my part, I've accepted responsibility for my shortcomings and apologize to myself.
333. The difficulties I face force me to develop as a person.
334. No changes need to be made to me because I am perfect as I am.
335. Learning from my errors aids my development.

336.   Things are looking up for today.
337.   The confidence and bravery I possess is unwavering.
338.   The level of joy I experience is entirely under my control.
339.   I am surrounded by people who adore and value me.
340.   I'm not afraid to fight for my convictions.
341.   The things I hope to accomplish inspire me.
342.   It's fine to admit ignorance sometimes.
343.   I'm going to try to have a good attitude today.
344.   Everything will not break me.
345.   If I set my mind to it, I can accomplish any goal.
346.   To exercise personal agency, I now grant myself permission.
347.   Next time, I'll be more prepared.
348.   Right now, I don't need anything else.
349.   I can accomplish a lot.
350.   There is no need to worry; everything will be fine.
351.   When I say something, I mean it.
352.   To put it simply, I am pleased with my own accomplishments.
353.   I have earned the right to joy.
354.   Yes, I can choose whatever I want to do.
355.   I am deserving of love.
356.   Yes, I can affect change.
357.   To put it simply, I am going to be confident today.
358.   For the first time in my life, I feel in control.

359. To make my goals a reality is within my control.
360. To put it simply, I have faith in my own skills and abilities.
361. I believe only good things are in store for me.
362. It is important that I exist.
363. As soon as I leave the house, I feel a surge of self-assurance.
364. outside my normal routine.
365. The more I think positively, the more positively
366. feelings.
367. I'm going to face my fears head-on today.
368. I'm eager to take in new information.
369. Each day is a new beginning.
370. Even if I do fail, I know I can always try again.
371. All of the pieces of me fit together perfectly.
372. The only person I can honestly judge my progress against is myself.
373. I'm capable of anything.
374. Putting forth my best effort is sufficient.
375. What I am depends entirely on my own imagination.
376. For the most part, I'm happy with myself.
377. That's right, folks; today is going to be one fantastic day.
378. Mistakes can and should be made.
379. The decisions I've been making have all been excellent ones.
380. It's important to me to be around upbeat, encouraging people.

381. The choices I've made have shaped who I am today.
382. As for me, I'm tough and persistent.
383. I'm finally going to have a good day today.
384. My true beauty lies within.
385. I am able to rely on my own strength.
386. Despite the difficulty, I will succeed.
387. Being present in the now is something I am capable of doing.
388. The first step in my process is to adopt an optimistic outlook.
389. The sky's the limit.
390. Positive vibes just seem to emanate from me.
391. Amazing things are on the horizon for
392. me.
393. I feel comfortable taking a few deep breaths.
394. Inhaling deeply, I am fortified.
395. I've got a fresh take on things, man.
396. Nothing but blessings should come my way.
397. The door to my future success is about to open.
398. I allow myself to be imperfect.
399. Present day is something for which I am grateful.
400. Each and every day, I work hard to give it my all.
401. I'm going to force myself to do it.
402. I can handle this.
403. I am capable of approaching the problem methodically.
404. I've decided to work at my own pace.
405. To put it simply, I'm going to gamble.

406. Today is my day to shine.
407. I will prevail over this challenge.
408. I'm going to make today fantastic.
409. My feelings are under my control.
410. The scope of my abilities is limitless.
411. I've settled into a peaceful state.
412. My current project is improving myself.
413. My mindset is set for victory.
414. On the inside and out, I am a stunning woman.
415. It's all good now.
416. My opinion counts.
417. Just as I am, is good enough for me.
418. I am making plans for the future.
419. As for me, I'm going to focus on the bright side.
420. To what extent I am happy depends on me.
421. I'm turning a new page in my life right now.
422. Regarding my judgment, I am confident.
423. I have the power to alter the course of history.
424. Clearly, I have a high IQ.
425. To have a positive or negative outlook is a decision I make for myself.
426. My presence is crucial.
427. I am on the path to perfection.
428. As for me, I intend to be an agent of good today.
429. More I let go, the better I'll feel.
430. I lay the groundwork and select the furniture for my own life.
431. I have so much vitality and happiness today.

432. My immune system is strong, my brain is sharp, and my spirit is at peace.
433. I have the power to rise above my inferior thoughts and deeds.
434. I have been bestowed with inexhaustible abilities, which I will now begin to exercise.
435. Those who have wronged me in the past have my forgiveness, and I now release all ties to them.
436. A flood of empathy washes away my hostility and is replaced by unconditional love.
437. It's not hard to see that I have what it takes to make it to the top of my field.
438. Inspiring creative juices flow through me, and I find myself having epiphanic insights.
439. Choose happiness. The things I have accomplished and the gifts I have received are the foundations upon which I build my sense of contentment.
440. My potential for success is boundless, and my ability to overcome adversity is unbounded.
441. I have guts and I speak up for what I believe in.
442. My mind is brimming with optimism, and good fortune has showered my life.
443. I'm giving up all my bad practices and replacing them with new, better ones today.
444. To put it simply, I am held in high esteem by those around me.
445. The people in my life are incredible, and I count myself very lucky.

446.   My sense of self-worth is through the roof, and I am full of confidence as a result.
447.   This whole thing is working out for my highest good.
448.   I am a juggernaut; no force on earth can stop me.
449.   Although this is a trying time, it is only temporary.
450.   The future I imagine for myself now is the best possible version of the future.
451.   Everything I do is backed up by the cosmos; I can literally see my goals coming to fruition.
452.   The beauty, charm, and grace that emanates from me is undeniable.
453.   I am winning this battle against my illness; I am getting stronger by the day.
454.   The roadblocks in my way are disappearing, and I can see the path of greatness ahead of me.
455.   This morning, I've got a lot of fire in my belly and a clear head.
456.   No matter what the future holds, I am content with the past and present.
457.   A new chapter in my life is opening up right now.
458.   I have courage.
459.   In the face of adversity, I boldly attempt to better myself.
460.   In other words, I am in tune with my feelings.
461.   The masculine and feminine aspects of my nature are in harmony.
462.   That's it, I give up and let the universe take care of me.

463. The feelings I have are valid.
464. I deserve to be loved, and I know it.
465. Quite simply, I adore myself.
466. To put it simply, I bounce back quickly.
467. My mindset is something I can adjust.
468. I am helpless in the face of opposition.
469. I can think things through and decide wisely on my own.
470. The tools I need to make today count are both within my grasp and within my mind and body.
471. I recognize that I am adequate, always have been, and always will be.
472. Every day that I am able to let go of my lingering self-doubt and negativity about my life, my self-confidence grows. What is good, I accept.
473. Through following my gut, I find myself led down ever-more-promising avenues of exploration daily. I have the ability to make sound choices
474. I accept all the good that is and will be coming into my life; I am living up to my full potential; I am focused and feel passionate about my work; I am motivated and work well under pressure;
475. To overcome any difficulty, I have everything I need.
476. I have the ability to grow in ways that will ultimately bring me fulfillment, independence, and satisfaction.
477. I consider myself extremely fortunate to have woken up to such a promising day.
478. I accept myself exactly as I am, and that's enough to make me happy.

479. Because I never stop thinking about and working on new ideas, my life is rich with possibilities for development.

480. The tough times I've had to endure have given me the chance to mature and develop as a person.

481. My life is a creation of my own design. I am laying the groundwork for it and picking out high-quality materials now.

482. I choose to better my mental and physical health today by letting go of negative routines and replacing them with new, more productive ones. I will live in the moment and savor each experience.

483. Today I will be a better person; one who is kinder, wiser, and more compassionate; one who gladly and completely fulfills the obligations that are placed upon me; one who is surrounded by supportive, loving people; one who is capable of making important decisions based

484. Peace, love, and prosperity are all in store for you today.

485. The money just keeps coming in.

486. To me, all of the riches of the universe come easily.

487. Affluence is something I am now willing to accept without hesitation, difficulty, or restraint.

488. The source of my wealth is boundless and overflowing, and for that I am eternally grateful.

489. When I put my hands on something, good fortune follows.

490. I attract wealth like a magnet.

491. Debt-free here I am.

492.   Happiness and prosperity are everywhere in my life.

493.   My requirements have been fulfilled in full.

494.   Success has found me.

495.   The money comes easily to me, and I have many sources of income.

496.   I am a generous giver as well as a gracious receiver.

497.   I've hit the jackpot and am floating downstream.

498.   When the Universe showers me with riches and joy, I gladly accept them.

499.   Finances have opened up for me in unexpected ways.

500.   Money is good to me, and I am good to money.

501.   As of right now, I am receiving an abundance of money.

502.   People are always giving me cash.

503.   Find me, and you'll find a priceless treasure.

504.   To my amazement, I have found a way to effortlessly attract an endless supply of money and

505.   prosperity into each and every one of my spheres of existence.

506.   For any situation, I can easily come up with the necessary funds.

507.   It seems that cash is coming my way from both expected and unexpected sources.

508.   In my life, cash flows freely, and there is always some to spare.

509.   I'm getting all the money I need.

510.   I no longer have to worry about money.

511.   To put it simply, cash is raining down on me.
512.   Funds are now flowing to me in ideal quantities and forms.
513.   There is an abundance of good in my life, in myself, and in everyone around me.
514.   Despite what others may think, I am able to see through deception and know that success is mine.
515.   I no longer have any financial obligations.
516.   I have been steadily increasing my earnings.
517.   I have an overabundance of creative energy.
518.   Everything I want or need can be bought with the money I have.
519.   Day after day, I receive monetary support.
520.   The monetary resources are readily available.
521.   In shape and physically appealing, that's me.
522.   Each day I am more prosperous.
523.   On the inside and out, I am a stunning woman.
524.   My daily weight loss goals are achievable.
525.   I make sure I get enough rest and eat healthily.
526.   Now my breaths are longer, deeper, and more at ease.
527.   My body is cherished and cared for by me, and I do the same for it.
528.   I'm a pretty girl.
529.   I have a lot of charm.
530.   At this moment, I feel calm and at ease.
531.   When I'm calm, my body is able to heal quickly from damage.

532. It's not just my physical appearance, but also my personality and character that make me attractive.

533. I go to bed early and get up bright and early.

534. My life is becoming a source of healing energy.

535. Today, I am whole and content.

536. The highest state of health and vitality is being manifested by me at this time.

537. At this very moment, I am whole and complete in every way—mentally, physically, spiritually, financially, and emotionally.

538. Now, I am able to keep my weight where it needs to be with relative ease.

539. My health and well-being are in my own hands.

540. The physical form that I have was given to me by God, and I am grateful.

541. I'm a very active person with a ton of stamina.

542. My complexion is healthy and glowing.

543. I've never had any trouble staying at a healthy weight.

544. The physical, mental, and spiritual parts of me are all fine.

545. I am a highly effective, highly energetic, physically fit woman who can easily deal with any situation that may arise right now.

546. I plan to work out for 15 minutes a day.

547. My spirit is high and my energy levels are high right now.

548. These days, I really look forward to eating my healthy, nutritious meals.

549.   If I want to improve my health, I can do it.

550.   In order to keep my body in tip-top shape, I enjoy working out and eating right.

551.   My mental, physical, and spiritual well-being are all at peak performance.

552.   The foods I eat are both healthy and nutritious.

553.   Nowadays, I look forward to my daily workouts.

554.   As an athlete, I am in good shape.

555.   I try to work out on a consistent basis.

556.   All of my internal organs are fully functional, and my body is healthy overall.

557.   It's safe to say that I enjoy good health and fitness.

558.   With each passing day, I inch closer to my goal weight.

559.   When my body requires energy, that's all I eat.

Final Thoughts

Affirmations in the morning might help us connect with our spirit. These are the most stimulating ways to start our days off well.

These not only assist us in overcoming self-defeating ideas and procrastination, but also encourage us to maximize our abilities, sharpen our talents, and achieve our goals.

My Kings, believe me when I say that these ultimate morning affirmations are your treasure chest for kicking off your days in the greatest possible way.

Let's make a conscious effort to repeat these affirmations in order to enhance our confidence and love our flaws.

Don't forget to leave a comment in the review box with your favorite powerful morning quote.

THE END

Thank you for taking the time to read the book! Your opinion matters, and your feedback can help other readers discover and enjoy the book as well. If you found value in this story, I kindly request that you share your thoughts and impressions by leaving a review on Amazon. Your review will not only support the author but also guide potential readers in making their decision. Simply click on the following link to share your review:

https://www.amazon.com/review/create-review/?ie=UTF8&channel=glance-detail&asin=B0BF3885D1

Thank you once again for your time, and I hope your review reflects the enjoyment you experienced while reading the book. Happy reviewing!

Made in the USA
Coppell, TX
22 September 2023